I0423580

DIABETIC DESSERT COOKBOOK

Top 60 Diabetic Dessert Recipes
(With Nutritional Values For Each Recipe)

BY
KATYA JOHANSSON

Contents

INTRODUCTION

Thank you for purchasing this cookbook I hope it will answer all your questions on diabetic dessert recipes. Diabetes can be a severe and debilitating condition. For those suffering from this disease, the right diet is imperative. This cookbook contains a healthy collection of dessert recipes that are diabetic friendly.

These recipes will keep you on the right track for controlling this disease and living a healthy lifestyle. Many people assume that once one has diabetes, then they must be on a strict diet that is tedious and painful to keep this disease in check. It is not true! As you will find out, the recipes in this book are just as delicious as any other non-diabetic recipes.

CHAPTER 1: DIABETIC-FRIENDLY FRUIT JAM DESSERT RECIPES

1. MANGO JAM

Ingredients:

- ¼ cup water
- One lime, freshly squeezed
- ¾ cup honey
- Four ripe mangoes, flesh diced
- Pinch of sea salt

Directions:

1. In a saucepan set over medium heat, combine water, lime, honey, mangoes, and salt. Bring to a boil. Reduce heat to low setting.
2. Using a wooden spoon, mash apricots. Stirring until liquid has evaporated.
3. Turn off the heat. Let cool at room temperature before storing in an airtight jar/container. Use as needed.

Nutritional Information

Calories: 110
Total Fat: 5 g
Total Carbohydrate: 17 g
Sugars: 7 g
Protein: 2 g
Sodium: 35 g

2. MANGO CINNAMON JAM

Ingredients:

- ¼ cup water
- ½ lemon, freshly squeezed
- 1 cup raw organic honey
- Two teaspoons cinnamon powder
- Four ripe mangoes, flesh diced
- Pinch of sea salt

Directions:

1. In a saucepan set over medium heat, combine water, lemon, honey, cinnamon powder, mangoes, and salt. Bring to a boil. Reduce heat to low setting.
2. Using a wooden spoon, mash mangoes.Stirring until liquid has evaporated.
3. Turn off the heat. Let cool at room temperature before storing in an airtight jar/container. Use as needed.

Nutritional Information

Calories: 100
Total Fat: 4 g
Total Carbohydrate: 18g
Sugars: 6 g
Protein: 2 g
Sodium: 30 g

3. APPLE JAM

Ingredients:

- ¼ cup water
- One lime, freshly squeezed
- ¾ cup honey
- Two apples, coarsely chopped
- Pinch of sea salt

Directions:

1. In a saucepan set over medium heat, combine water, lime, honey, apples, and salt. Bring to a boil. Reduce heat to low setting.
2. Using a wooden spoon, mash apricots. Stirring until liquid has evaporated.
3. Turn off the heat. Let cool at room temperature before storing in an airtight jar/container. Use as needed.

Nutritional Information

Calories: 90
Total Fat: 4 g
Total Carbohydrate: 11 g
Sugars: 5g
Protein: 1 g
Sodium: 23 g

4. APPLE CINNAMON JAM

Ingredients:

- ¼ cup water
- ½ lemon, freshly squeezed
- 1 cup raw organic honey
- Two teaspoons cinnamon powder
- Two apples, coarsely chopped
- Pinch of sea salt

Directions:

1. In a saucepan set over medium heat, combine water, lemon, honey, cinnamon powder, apples, and salt. Bring to a boil. Reduce heat to low setting.
2. Using a wooden spoon, mash apples. Stirring frequently until liquid has evaporated.
3. Turn off the heat. Let cool at room temperature before storing in an airtight jar/container. Use as needed.

Nutritional Information

Calories: 67
   Total Fat: 5 g
   Total Carbohydrate: 18 g
   Sugars: 9 g
   Protein: 2 g
   Sodium: 23 g

5. CHERRY JAM

Ingredients:

- ¼ cup water
- ½ lemon, freshly squeezed
- 1 cup raw organic honey
- 2 cups cherries, halved
- Pinch of sea salt

Directions:

1. In a saucepan set over medium heat, combine water, lemon, honey, cherries, and salt. Bring to a boil. Reduce heat to low setting.
2. Using a wooden spoon, mash apricots. Stirring frequently until liquid has evaporated.
3. Turn off the heat. Let cool at room temperature before storing in an airtight jar/container. Use as needed.

Nutritional Information

Calories: 110
Total Fat: 5 g
Total Carbohydrate: 17 g
Sugars: 7 g
Protein: 2 g
Sodium: 35 g

6. CHERRY CINNAMON JAM

Ingredients:

- ¼ cup water
- ½ lemon, freshly squeezed
- 1 cup raw organic honey
- Two teaspoons cinnamon powder
- 2 cups cherries, halved
- Pinch of sea salt

Directions:

1. In a saucepan set over medium heat, combine water, lemon, honey, cinnamon powder, cherries, and salt. Bring to a boil. Reduce heat to low setting.
2. Using a wooden spoon, mash cherries. Stirring frequently until liquid has evaporated.
3. Turn off the heat. Let cool at room temperature before storing in an airtight jar/container. Use as needed.

Nutritional Information

Calories: 88
Total Fat: 3 g
Total Carbohydrate: 8 g
Sugars: 9 g
Protein: 2 g
Sodium: 34 g

7. PEACH JAM

Ingredients:

- ¼ cup water
- ½ lemon, freshly squeezed juice
- 1 cup raw organic honey
- Two peaches, cubed
- Pinch of sea salt

Directions:

1. In a saucepan set over medium heat, combine water, lemon, honey, peaches, and salt. Bring to a boil. Reduce heat to low setting.
2. Using a wooden spoon, mash peaches. Stirring frequently until liquid has evaporated.
3. Turn off the heat. Let cool at room temperature before storing in an airtight jar/container. Use as needed.

Nutritional Information

Calories: 110
Total Fat: 5 g
Total Carbohydrate: 17 g
Sugars: 7 g
Protein: 2 g
Sodium: 35 g

8. Peach Cinnamon Jam

Ingredients:

- ¼ cup water
- ½ lemon, freshly squeezed
- 1 cup raw organic honey
- 2 teaspoons cinnamon powder
- 2 peaches, cubed
- Pinch of sea salt

Directions:

1. In a saucepan set over medium heat, combine water, lemon, honey, cinnamon powder, peaches, and salt. Bring to a boil. Reduce heat to low setting.
2. Using a wooden spoon, mash peaches. Stirring frequently until liquid has evaporated.
3. Turn off the heat. Let cool at room temperature before storing in an airtight jar/container. Use as needed.

Nutritional Information

Calories: 87
Total Fat: 3 g
Total Carbohydrate: 10 g
Sugars: 6 g
Protein: 3 g
Sodium: 30g

9. PINEAPPLE JAM

Ingredients:

- ¼ cup water
- Two lime, freshly squeezed
- 1 cup raw organic honey
- One fresh pineapple, pulp diced
- Pinch of sea salt

Directions:

1. In a saucepan set over medium heat, combine water, lime, honey, pineapple, and salt. Bring to a boil. Reduce heat to low setting.
2. Using a wooden spoon, mash pineapple. Stirring frequently until liquid has evaporated.
3. Turn off the heat. Let cool at room temperature before storing in an airtight jar/container. Use as needed.

Nutritional Information

Calories: 110
Total Fat: 5 g
Total Carbohydrate: 17 g
Sugars: 7 g
Protein: 2 g
Sodium: 35 g

10. PLUM JAM

Ingredients:

- ¼ cup water
- ½ lemon, freshly squeezed
- 1 cup raw organic honey
- 2 lbs plums, diced
- Pinch of sea salt

Directions:

1. In a saucepan set over medium heat, combine water, lemon, honey, plums, and salt. Bring to a boil. Reduce heat to low setting.
2. Using a wooden spoon, mash plum. Stirring frequently until liquid has evaporated.
3. Turn off the heat. Let cool at room temperature before storing in an airtight jar/container. Use as needed.

Nutritional Information

Calories: 50
Total Fat: 4 g
Total Carbohydrate: 12 g
Sugars: 6 g
Protein: 1 g
Sodium: 20 g

11. EASY STRAWBERRY JAM

Ingredients:

- 2½ cups frozen strawberries, thawed
- 1 cup raw organic honey
- ¼ cup water
- ½ lemon, freshly squeezed
- Pinch of sea salt

Directions:

1. In a saucepan set over medium heat, combine water, lemon, honey, plums, and salt. Bring to a boil. Reduce heat to low setting.
2. Using a wooden spoon, mash strawberry. Stirring frequently until liquid has evaporated.
3. Turn off the heat. Let cool at room temperature before storing in an airtight jar/container. Use as needed.

Nutritional Information

Calories: 110
Total Fat: 5 g
Total Carbohydrate: 17 g
Sugars: 7 g
Protein: 2 g
Sodium: 35 g

12. RASPBERRY JAM

Ingredients:

- ¼ cup water
- ½ lemon, freshly squeezed
- 1 cup raw organic honey
- 2½ lbs frozen raspberries, thawed
- Pinch of sea salt

Directions:

1. In a saucepan set over medium heat, combine water, lemon, honey, raspberries, and salt. Bring to a boil. Reduce heat to low setting.
2. Using a wooden spoon, mash raspberries. Stirring frequently until liquid has evaporated.
3. Turn off the heat. Let cool at room temperature before storing in an airtight jar/container. Use as needed.

Nutritional Information

Calories: 78
Total Fat: 5 g
Total Carbohydrate: 19g
Sugars: 9 g
Protein: 3 g
Sodium: 37 g

13. RASPBERRY JAM WITH CHIA SEEDS

Ingredients:

- 1 cup raw organic honey
- 3 cups fresh raspberries
- ¼ cup water
- Two tablespoons chia seeds
- One tablespoon lemon juice, fresh squeezed

Directions:

1. In a saucepan set over medium heat, combine honey and raspberries. Bring to a boil. Reduce heat to low setting. Add water, lemon juice, and chia seeds.
2. Using a potato masher, mash the raspberries. Stirring frequently until liquid has evaporated.
3. Turn off the heat. Let cool at room temperature before storing in an airtight jar/container. Use as needed.

Nutritional Information

Calories: 110
    Total Fat: 5 g
    Total Carbohydrate: 17 g
    Sugars: 7 g
    Protein: 2 g
    Sodium: 35 g

14. STRAWBERRY JAM WITH FLAX SEEDS

Ingredients:

- 1 cup raw organic honey
- 1 lb frozen strawberries, thawed
- ¼ cup water
- One tablespoon lemon juice, freshly squeezed
- Two tablespoons flaxseeds

Directions:

1. In a saucepan set over medium heat, combine honey and fruits. Bring to a boil. Reduce heat to low setting. Add water, lemon juice, and flaxseeds.
2. Using a potato masher, mash the raspberries. Stirring frequently until liquid has evaporated.
3. Turn off the heat. Let cool at room temperature before storing in an airtight jar/container. Use as needed.

Nutritional Information

Calories: 100
Total Fat: 4 g
Total Carbohydrate: 13 g
Sugars: 6 g
Protein: 3 g
Sodium: 30 g

15. VANILLA BERRY OVERLOAD

Ingredients:

- ¼ cup water
- 1 cup raw organic honey
- ½ lemon, freshly squeezed
- 1 cup frozen cranberries, thawed
- 1 cup frozen blackberries, thawed
- 1 cup frozen blueberries, thawed
- One vanilla pod, halved lengthwise
- Pinch of sea salt

Directions:

1. In a saucepan set over medium heat, combine water, honey lemon, cranberries, blackberries, blueberries, vanilla pod, and salt.
2. Using a potato masher, mash the berries. Stirring frequently until liquid has evaporated.
3. Turn off the heat. Let cool at room temperature before storing in an airtight jar/container. Use as needed.

Nutritional Information

Calories: 110
Total Fat: 5 g
Total Carbohydrate: 17 g
Sugars: 7 g
Protein: 2 g
Sodium: 35 g

CHAPTER 2: NUT AND SEED BUTTERS AND CHEESES

16. PECAN-ALMOND BUTTER

Ingredients:

- ¾ cup raw pecans, chopped
- 1 cup raw blanched almond slivers
- One vanilla pod, halved lengthwise
- One tablespoon raw organic honey
- ¼ teaspoon sea salt

Directions:

1. Preheat the oven to 350°F.
2. Line a baking sheet with aluminium foil. Spread nuts on the baking sheet. Bake for 10 minutes or until golden brown.
3. Remove from heat. Cool before placing into a food processor. Add vanilla pod, honey, and salt. Process until smooth. Store in airtight container.

Nutritional Information

Calories: 123
Total Fat: 4 g
Total Carbohydrate: 19 g
Sugars: 6g
Protein: 3 g
Sodium: 43 g

17. Coconut-Cashew Butter with Sesame Seeds

Ingredients:

- 2 tablespoons sesame seeds
- 1½ cups raw cashew nuts halved
- ½ cup coconut flakes, unsweetened
- One tablespoon coconut oil
- ¼ teaspoon sea salt

Directions:

1. Preheat the oven to 350°F.
2. Line a baking sheet with aluminium foil. Spread sesame seeds nuts, coconut flakes, and cashew nuts on the baking sheet. Bake for 10 minutes or until golden brown.
3. Remove from heat. Cool before placing into a food processor. Pour olive oil and salt. Process until smooth. Store in airtight container.

Nutritional Information

Calories: 110
Total Fat: 5 g
Total Carbohydrate: 17 g
Sugars: 7 g
Protein: 2 g
Sodium: 35 g

18. Coconut Butter

Ingredients:
- 4 cups coconut flakes, unsweetened

Directions:
1. Process coconut flakes in a blender until smooth
2. Store in airtight container; use as needed.

Nutritional Information
Calories: 134
Total Fat: 7 g
Total Carbohydrate: 9g
Sugars: 5 g
Protein: 2 g
Sodium: 24 g

19. Coconut and Honey Butter

Ingredients:

- ⅛ teaspoon raw organic honey
- 4 cups coconut flakes, unsweetened
- pinch of sea salt

Directions:

1. Process honey, coconut flakes, and salt in a blender until smooth
2. Store in airtight container; use as needed.

Nutritional Information

Calories: 110
Total Fat: 5 g
Total Carbohydrate: 17 g
Sugars: 7 g
Protein: 2 g
Sodium: 35 g

20. BASIC ALMOND CHEESE

Ingredients:

- One teaspoon lemon juice, freshly squeezed
- 1 cup blanched almonds, soaked in water overnight
- ⅛ teaspoon sea salt
- 2 cups water, filtered
- raw organic honey for drizzling

Directions:

1. In a food processor, combine lemon juice, almonds, and salt. Pour water and process until smooth.
2. Drape cheesecloth into fine-meshed. Pour in mixture to drain. Tie cheesecloth into a knot. Gently squeeze out liquids. Set aside for 1 day.
3. **Place cheese in the fridge for 1 hour to set. Remove cheesecloth. Slice cheese.**

Nutritional Information

Calories: 98
Total Fat: 7 g
Total Carbohydrate: 10 g
Sugars: 6 g
Protein: 4 g
Sodium: 21g

21. Basic Cashew Cheese

Ingredients:

- 1 cup raw cashew nuts, soaked in water overnight
- 1 teaspoon lemon juice, fresh squeezed, pips removed
- ⅛ teaspoon sea salt
- 2 cups water, filtered

Same preparation method as Basic Almond Cheese

Nutritional Information

Calories: 110
Total Fat: 5 g
Total Carbohydrate: 17 g
Sugars: 7 g
Protein: 2 g
Sodium: 35 g

22. Basic Pecan Cheese

Ingredients:

- 1 cup raw pecan nuts, soaked in water overnight
- One teaspoon lemon juice, fresh squeezed
- ⅛ teaspoon sea salt
- 2 cups water, filtered
- One fresh apricot, diced for garnish

Same preparation method as Basic Almond Cheese

Nutritional Information

Calories: 89
Total Fat: 6 g
Total Carbohydrate: 12g
Sugars: 5 g
Protein: 4 g
Sodium: 39 g

Nutritional Information

Calories: 110
Total Fat: 5 g
Total Carbohydrate: 17 g
Sugars: 7 g
Protein: 2 g
Sodium: 35 g

23. BASIC MACADAMIA CHEESE

Ingredients:

- 1 cup raw macadamia nuts, soaked in water overnight
- One teaspoon lemon juice, freshly squeezed
- ⅛ teaspoon sea salt
- 2 cups water, filtered
- dried basil leaves, for sprinkling

Same preparation method as Basic Almond Cheese

Nutritional Information

Calories: 98
Total Fat: 6 g
Total Carbohydrate: 11 g
Sugars: 6 g
Protein: 5 g
Sodium: 32 g

24. Basic Walnut Cheese

Ingredients:

- 1 cup raw walnuts, soaked in water overnight
- 1 teaspoon lemon juice, freshly squeezed
- ⅛ teaspoon sea salt
- 2 cups water, filtered
- One pear, thinly sliced

Same preparation method as Basic Almond Cheese

Nutritional Information

Calories: 110
Total Fat: 5 g
Total Carbohydrate: 17 g
Sugars: 7 g
Protein: 2 g
Sodium: 35 g

24. SPICY CASHEW BUTTER WITH FLAXSEEDS

Ingredients:

- 1 cup coconut milk
- One tablespoon coconut oil, melted
- Onecan sweet potato puree
- Two tablespoons raw organic honey
- 1 cup raw cashew nuts, soaked in water overnight
- Two tablespoons flaxseed meal
- Two large vanilla pods halved lengthwise
- 1½ teaspoon all spice powder
- ¼ teaspoon nutmeg powder
- ½ teaspoon ginger powder
- Pinch of sea salt

Directions:

1. Place coconut milk, coconut oil, sweet potato puree, honey, cashew nuts, flaxseed meal, vanilla pods, allspice powder, nutmeg, ginger, and salt into food processor.
2. Process until smooth. Transfer into anairtight container. Use as needed.

Nutritional Information

Calories: 123
Total Fat: 6 g
Total Carbohydrate: 21 g
Sugars: 8 g
Protein: 7 g
Sodium: 35g

25. SPICY PECAN BUTTER WITH CHIA SEEDS

Ingredients:

- 1 cup coconut milk
- One tablespoon coconut oil, melted
- One can, sweet potato puree
- Three tablespoons raw organic honey
- 1 cup raw pecans, soaked in water overnight
- Two tablespoon chia seeds
- Two vanilla pods, halved lengthwise
- 1½ teaspoon cinnamon powder
- ½ teaspoon ginger powder
- ¼ teaspoon nutmeg powder
- Pinch of salt

Directions:

1. Place coconut milk, coconut oil, sweet potato puree, honey, pecans, chia seeds, vanilla pods, cinnamon powder, ginger powder, nutmeg, and salt into food processor.
2. Process until smooth. Transfer into anairtight container. Use as needed.

Nutritional Information

Calories: 110
Total Fat: 5 g
Total Carbohydrate: 17 g
Sugars: 7 g
Protein: 2 g
Sodium: 35 g

26. SUNFLOWER SEED BUTTER

Ingredients:
- 3 cups raw sunflower seeds
- ¼ cup raw organic honey
- Two tablespoons coconut oil, melted
- One vanilla pod, halved lengthwise
- ½ teaspoon cinnamon powder
- Pinch of sea salt

Same preparation method as Coconut Butter

Nutritional Information

Calories: 110
Total Fat: 5 g
Total Carbohydrate: 17 g
Sugars: 7 g
Protein: 2 g
Sodium: 35 g

27. SWEET POTATO BUTTER WITH DRIED CRANBERRIES

Ingredients:
- Three tablespoons raw organic honey
- One can sweet potato puree
- ⅛ teaspoon apple cider vinegar
- ¼ cup dried cranberries
- pinch of sea salt
- dash of all spice powder
- pinch of cinnamon powder
- bit of cumin powder
- pinch of ginger powder

Same preparation method as**Coconut Butter**

Place ingredients into food processor. Pulse/process to mix, scraping down sides of container often. Butter should be chunky but spreadable. If not, add more apple cider vinegar; pulse after each addition. Transfer butter into anairtight container; use as needed.

Nutritional Information
Calories: 97
Total Fat: 4 g
Total Carbohydrate: 12 g
Sugars: 5 g
Protein: 4 g
Sodium: 36 g

CHAPTER 3: DIABETIC-FRIENDLY MUFFIN DESSERTS AND BREAD

28. Blueberry and Lemon Muffins

Ingredients:

- 1½ cup fresh blueberries, rinsed

Dry ingredients

- 1½ teaspoons baking soda
- 2 cups unbleached all-purpose flour
- 2 teaspoons fresh lemon zest
- ½ teaspoons kosher salt
- One tablespoon freshly squeezed lemon juice
- 1 cup low-fat milk
- ¾ cup maple syrup
- 1/3 cup coconut oil

Directions:

1. Preheat oven to 375°F.
2. Place paper liners into muffin tins. Combine baking soda, all-purpose flour, lemon zest, and salt. Mix well.
3. In another bowl, combine lemon juice, milk, maple syrup, and oil. Pour wet ingredients over dry ingredients. Stir well.
4. Fold in blueberries. Spoon equal portions into lined muffin depressions.
5. Bake for 25 minutes or until toothpick comes out clean. Remove from oven. Cool cupcakes. Serve.

Nutritional Information

Calories: 110
Total Fat: 5 g
Total Carbohydrate: 17 g
Sugars: 7 g
Protein: 2 g

Sodium: 35 g

29. CARROTS AND CASHEW MUFFINS

Ingredients:

- 1½ cups whole wheat pastry flour
- Two teaspoons baking soda
- Four large carrots, shredded
- Two servings flax eggs
- ½ cup steel-cut oats
- ½ cup brown sugar
- ¼ cup coconut oil
- One teaspoon vanilla extract
- ¼ cup cashew nuts, chopped

Directions:

1. Preheat oven to 375°F.
2. Place paper liners into muffin tins. Combine pastry flour, baking soda, carrots, flax eggs, oats, and brown sugar, oil, vanilla extract, and cashew nuts. Do not over mix.
3. Spoon batter into muffin depressions.
4. Bake for 20 minutes or until atoothpick inserted in centre comes out clean. Remove from oven. Allow cooling before serving.

Nutritional Information

Calories: 97
Total Fat: 4 g
Total Carbohydrate: 13 g
Sugars: 8 g
Protein: 9 g
Sodium: 43 g

30. Corn and Raspberry Muffins

Ingredients:

- 1¾ cup whole wheat pastry flour
- Two teaspoons baking powder
- 1 serving flax egg
- 1⅛ cup coconut milk
- ¼ cup coconut oil
- ½ cup fresh raspberries, rinsed, drained
- ¼ cup canned whole corn kernels, drained
- Three tablespoons brown sugar
- ½ teaspoon kosher salt

Direction:

1. Preheat oven to 375°F.
2. Place paper liners into muffin tins. Combine flour, baking powder, flax egg, coconut milk, coconut oil, raspberries, corn kernels, brown sugar and salt. Do not over mix.
3. Spoon batter into lined muffin depressions.
4. Bake for 20 minutes or until toothpick comes out clean. Remove from oven. Cool before removing muffins from tins. Allow cooling on cake rack. Serve.

Nutritional Information

Calories: 110
Total Fat: 5 g
Total Carbohydrate: 17 g
Sugars: 7 g
Protein: 2 g
Sodium: 35 g

31. CRANBERRY MUFFINS IN BLOOD ORANGE

Ingredients:

- 1¾ cup all-purpose flour
- Two teaspoons baking powder
- 1 serving flax egg
- 1 cup coconut milk
- ¼ cup coconut oil
- Three tablespoons sweet orange juice, freshly squeeze
- ½ cup fresh cranberries, drained
- ¼ cup shelled walnuts, roughly chopped
- Three tablespoons palm sugar, crumbled
- ½ teaspoon kosher salt

Directions:

1. Preheat the oven to 375°F.
2. Place paper liners into muffin tins. Combine flour, baking powder, flax egg, coconut milk, coconut oil, sweet orange juice, cranberries, walnuts, sugar, and salt. Do not over mix.
3. Spoon batter into lined muffin depressions.
4. Bake for 20 minutes or until toothpick comes out clean. Remove from oven. Allow cooling before removing muffins from tins. Place on a cake rack. Serve.

Nutritional Information

Calories: 110
Total Fat: 5 g
Total Carbohydrate: 17 g
Sugars: 7 g
Protein: 2 g
Sodium: 35 g

32. CRANBERRIES WITH WALNUTS MUFFINS

Ingredients:
- 1¾ cup all-purpose flour
- Two teaspoons baking powder
- 1 serving flax egg
- ¼ cup coconut oil
- 1⅛ cups walnut milk
- ¼ cup shelled walnuts, roughly chopped
- ½ cup fresh cranberries, drained
- Three tablespoons palm sugar, crumbled
- ½ teaspoon kosher salt

Directions:
1. Preheat oven to 375°F.
2. Place paper liners into muffin tins. Combine flour, baking powder, flax egg, coconut oil, walnut milk, walnuts, cranberries, palm sugar, and salt. Do not over mix.
3. Spoon batter into muffin depressions.
4. **Bake for 20 or until toothpick comes out clean. Remove from oven. Allow cooling before removing muffins from tins. Place on a cake rack. Serve.**

Nutritional Information
Calories: 87
Total Fat: 5 g
Total Carbohydrate: 19 g
Sugars: 5 g
Protein: 1 g
Sodium: 38 g

33. OATMEAL MUFFINS IN MAPLE SYRUP

Ingredients:

- 1½ cups whole wheat pastry flour
- One teaspoon baking powder
- One teaspoon baking soda
- ½ cup steel cut oats
- Two servings flax eggs
- 1¼ cups coconut milk
- ¼ cup coconut oil
- ¼ cup pure maple syrup
- One teaspoon vanilla extract
- ½ teaspoon kosher salt

Directions:

1. Preheat oven to 375°F.
2. Place paper liners into muffin tins. Combine flour, baking powder, baking soda, and oats. In another bowl, combine flax eggs, coconut milk, coconut oil, maple syrup, vanilla extract, and salt. Stir until well combined.
3. Spoon batter into muffin depressions.
4. Bake for 25 minutes or until toothpick comes out clean. Remove from oven. Cool cupcakes before serving.

Nutritional Information

Calories: 110
Total Fat: 5 g
Total Carbohydrate: 17 g
Sugars: 7 g
Protein: 2 g
Sodium: 35 g

34. RAISINS AND PLANTAIN MUFFINS

Ingredients:

- ¼ cup raisins
- 1½ cups whole wheat pastry flour
- Two teaspoons baking soda
- ½ cup steel-cut oats
- 2 servings flax eggs
- 4 pieces overripe plantains, mashed
- ½ cup palm sugar, crumbled
- ¼ cup coconut oil
- ¼ cup water
- One teaspoon vanilla extract

Directions:

1. Soak raisins in water for 2 hours before using.
2. Preheat the oven to 375°F. Place paper liners into muffin tins. Combine flour, baking soda, oats, flax eggs, plantains, sugar, coconut oil, water, and vanilla extract. Do not over mix.
3. Spoon batter into lined muffin depressions.
4. Bake for 15 minutes or until atoothpick inserted in centre comes out clean. Remove from oven. Cool cupcakes before serving.

Nutritional Information
Calories: 126
Total Fat: 4 g
Total Carbohydrate: 19 g
Sugars: 2 g
Protein: 2 g
Sodium: 21 g

35. ALMOND-COCONUT BREAD

Ingredients:
- coconut oil for greasing aloaf tin
- Four tablespoons coconut flour
- 4 cups almond flour
- One teaspoon baking soda
- ½ cup flaxseed meal
- ½ teaspoon sea salt
- Two tablespoons coconut vinegar
- Ten large eggs whisked

Directions:
1. Preheat the oven to 350°F.
2. Lightly grease loaf tin. Mix coconut flour, almond meal, baking soda, flaxseed meal, and salt. Make a well in the centre and pour coconut vinegar and eggs. Mix well until just combined. Pour batter into theloaf tin.
3. Bake for 35 minutes or until atoothpick inserted in centre comes out clean. Remove pan from oven. Allow cake to cool completely. Slice and serve plain or toasted.

Nutritional Information
Calories: 110
Total Fat: 5 g
Total Carbohydrate: 17 g
Sugars: 7 g
Protein: 2 g
Sodium: 35 g

36. BREAD STICKS SPRINKLED WITH CARAWAY SEEDS

Ingredients:

- One tablespoon black caraway seeds
- coconut oil for greasing

For the Bread

- 4 cups almond flour
- Four tablespoons ghee
- Four large eggs, whisked
- One teaspoon sea salt

Directions:

1. Preheat oven to 350°F.
2. Line baking sheets with aluminium foil. Lightly grease with oil.
3. Combine almond flour, ghee, eggs, and salt in a bowl. Mix until thedough comes together.
4. Place dough on thelightly floured surface and knead until elastic. Rest dough for 5 minutes, covered.
5. Roll dough and divide into balls. Roll each out into breadsticks and place on baking sheets.
6. Brush ghee on each stick. Sprinkle caraway seeds on top. Bake for 10 minutes.
7. Remove from oven. Let cool and serve.

Nutritional Information

Calories: 106
Total Fat: 5 g
Total Carbohydrate: 6 g
Sugars: 8 g
Protein: 3 g

Sodium: 20 g

37. Coconut Bread Sticks

Ingredients:

- coconut oil for greasing
- coconut flakes, unsweetened

For the Bread:

- Six tablespoons coconut flour
- 3 cups almond flour
- Four large eggs, whisked
- Four tablespoons ghee
- ½ teaspoon sea salt

Directions:

1. Preheat oven to 350°F/175°C. Line a baking sheet with aluminium foil. Grease with coconut oil.
2. In a bowl, combine coconut flour, almond meal, eggs, ghee, and salt. Mix until thedough comes together. Put dough on a floured surface. Knead until the dough is no longer sticky. Let dough rest for 5 minutes, covered.
3. Turn out thedough, roll into a log and divide into small balls. Then roll into sticks Roll each out into bread sticks. Place sticks on a baking sheet.
4. Brush each stick with ghee. Sprinkle with coconut flakes on top.
5. Bake for 10 minutes. Remove from the oven and let cool. Serve.

Nutritional Information

Calories: 110
Total Fat: 5 g
Total Carbohydrate: 17 g
Sugars: 7 g
Protein: 2 g

Sodium: 35 g

38. CHIA SEED BREAD

Ingredients:
- coconut oil for greasing
- 3 cups almond flour
- 1½ teaspoon baking soda
- ⅓ cup arrowroot powder
- ½ tablespoon chia seed, coarsely ground
- ½ teaspoon sea salt
- ¾ cup coconut cream
- Five eggs, whisked
- 1½ teaspoons coconut vinegar
- ½ cup butter, melted
- One teaspoon chia seeds, whole

Directions:
1. Preheat oven to 350°F.
2. Lightly grease loaf tin with coconut oil.
3. Combine almond flour, baking soda, cup arrowroot powder, ground chia seeds, and salt in a bowl. Make a well in the centre. Pour coconut cream, eggs, vinegar, and butter. Stir until well combined. Pour into theloaf tin. Sprinkle whole chia seeds on top.
4. Bake for 30 minutes or until atoothpick inserted in centre comes out clean. Remove from the oven and let cool. Serve.

Nutritional Information
Calories: 59
Total Fat: 9 g
Total Carbohydrate: 5 g
Sugars: 9 g
Protein: 9 g
Sodium: 26g

39. CHESTNUT BREAD

Ingredients:

- coconut oil for greasing
- 2 cups chestnut flour
- ²/₃ cup arrowroot flour
- 3 cups almond meal
- Two tablespoons coconut flakes, divided
- ½ cup roasted chestnuts, diced
- 1½ teaspoons sea salt
- ²/₃ cup coconut oil
- ²/₃ cup coconut cream
- Two tablespoons raw organic honey
- 14 large eggs, whites separated

Directions:

1. Preheat oven to 325°F.
2. Line a loaf tin with parchment paper and grease with coconut oil.
3. Combine chestnut flour, arrowroot flour, almond meal, coconut flakes, chestnuts, and sea salt. Make a well in the centre and pour coconut oil, coconut cream, and honey. Mix until well combined.
4. In another bowl, whisk egg whites until peaks form. Fold into bread batter. Pour batter into loaf tins. Sprinkle coconut flakes.
5. Bake for 40 minutes or until toothpick comes out clean. Allow cooling in tins for 1 hour. Place on a cake rack to cool completely. Serve.

Nutritional Information

Calories: 110
Total Fat: 5 g

Total Carbohydrate: 17 g
Sugars: 7 g
Protein: 2 g
Sodium: 35 g

40. RAISIN BREAD

Ingredients:
- ½ cup sultanas
- ½ cup raisins
- Two teaspoons nutmeg powder
- 1 cup almond flour
- Two teaspoons baking soda
- Two teaspoons cinnamon powder
- Two tablespoons lime juice, fresh squeezed
- Six pieces eggs whisked
- Two teaspoons vanilla extract
- Pinch sea salt
- water for soaking

Directions:
1. Soak raisins and sultanas in water until they double in size. Drain.
2. Preheat the oven to 350°F. Line loaf tin with parchment paper. Grease with coconut butter.
3. In a bowl, combine soaked sultanas and raisins, nutmeg powder, flour, baking soda, cinnamon powder, lime juice, eggs, vanilla extract, and salt. Mix until well combined. Pour batter into theloaf tin. Bake for 45 minutes.
4. Remove from the oven and place on a cake rack. Serve.

Nutritional Information
Calories: 99
Total Fat: 7 g
Total Carbohydrate: 18g
Sugars: 8 g
Protein: 9 g
Sodium: 28 g

41. NUTTY BREAD

Ingredients:

- One tablespoon pine nuts, chopped
- ½ teaspoon sesame seeds
- ½ teaspoon shelled roasted pumpkin seeds
- One tablespoon blanched almond slivers
- dash dried basil, shredded
- pinch dried thyme, shredded

For the bread loaf

- Four tablespoons coconut oil
- 1 cup almond flour
- 1 cup coconut flour
- Five large eggs, whisked
- ¼ cup tapioca flour
- One teaspoon baking soda
- One tablespoon coconut vinegar
- ¼ teaspoon sea salt

Directions:

1. Preheat the oven to 350°F.
2. Line a loaf tin with aluminium foil. Grease with coconut oil.
3. Combine almond flour, coconut flour, eggs, tapioca flour, baking soda, coconut vinegar, and salt. Pour batter into theloaf tin. Sprinkle with pine nuts, sesame seeds, almond slivers, dried basil, and dried thyme.
4. Bake for 30. Remove from heat and let cool for 1 hour. Place on a cake rack to cool completely. Serve.

Nutritional Information

Calories: 110
Total Fat: 5 g

Total Carbohydrate: 17 g
Sugars: 7 g
Protein: 2 g
Sodium: 35 g

42. Basil Pesto Bruschetta

Ingredients:

- Onetomato, halved
- 1 Kaiser roll halved lengthwise
- One tablespoon basil pesto sauce
- One tablespoon cashew cheese

Directions:

1. On a bread roll, spread pesto sauce and tomato slices. Drizzle cashew cheese on top.
2. Heat the bruschetta in a toaster until warmed through. Serve.

Nutritional Information

Calories: 78
Total Fat: 6 g
Total Carbohydrate: 11 g
Sugars: 8 g
Protein: 4 g
Sodium: 39 g

43. CHICKPEA SALAD SANDWICH

Ingredients:

- One slice whole wheat bread

For the chickpea salad

- ½ teaspoon Homemade Tahini
- ¼ cup avocado, mashed
- ¼ cup canned chickpeas, soft
- ¼ teaspoon fresh parsley, minced
- Pinch of kosher salt
- Pinch of white pepper

Directions:

1. In a mixing bowl, combine tahini, avocado, chickpea, parsley, salt, and pepper. Spread on top of the bread slice.
2. Heat the bruschetta in a toaster until warmed through. Serve.

Nutritional Information

Calories: 110
Total Fat: 5 g
Total Carbohydrate: 17 g
Sugars: 7 g
Protein: 2 g
Sodium: 35 g

44. Corn Hummus Sandwich

Ingredients:

- One slice whole wheat bread
- 1½ tablespoon hummus
- ½ tablespoon onion, diced
- One tablespoon whole corn kernels, canned
- ½ tablespoon green tomato, diced
- One tablespoon lime juice, freshly squeezed
- ½ tablespoon cilantro leaves, minced
- ⅛ teaspoon palm sugar, crumbled
- Pinch of sea salt

Directions:

1. Spread hummus on bread. Heat the bread in a toaster oven.
2. Meanwhile, in a mixing bowl, combine onion, corn kernels, tomatoes, lime juice, cilantro, palm sugar, and salt. Spread on top of the sandwich. Serve.

Nutritional Information

Calories: 98
Total Fat: 9 g
Total Carbohydrate: 17 g
Sugars: 6 g
Protein: 3 g
Sodium: 34 g

45. Mushroom Bruschetta

Ingredients:

- One slice whole wheat bread
- One tablespoon basil-cashew pesto sauce
- One teaspoon olive oil
- One large porcini mushroom, thinly sliced
- One garlic clove, minced
- One teaspoon parsley, minced
- One tablespoon balsamic vinegar
- Pinch of salt
- One teaspoon palm sugar

Directions:

1. Spread basil-cashew pesto sauce on one side of the bread. Set aside.
2. Meanwhile, in a skillet over medium heat, saute mushrooms. Add garlic, parsley, balsamic vinegar, salt, and sugar. Stir well.
3. Let it simmer for 5 minutes. Remove from heat.
4. Spoon mixture ad spread on top of the bread. Serve.

Nutritional Information

Calories: 110
Total Fat: 5 g
Total Carbohydrate: 17 g
Sugars: 7 g
Protein: 2 g
Sodium: 35 g

46. MUSHROOMS BRUSCHETTA ON HUMMUS

Ingredients:

- One slice toasted Coriander Bread
- ½ tablespoon Hummus
- ¼ teaspoon coriander, minced
- ½ cup canned straw mushrooms halved
- ½ tablespoon cashew cheese
- Pinch of kosher salt
- Pinch of white pepper

Directions:

1. In a bowl, combine hummus, coriander, straw mushrooms, and cashew cheese. Season with salt and pepper.
2. Spread on top of bread. Heat in a toaster oven. Serve.

Nutritional Information

Calories: 145
Total Fat: 5 g
Total Carbohydrate: 19 g
Sugars: 6 g
Protein: 4 g
Sodium: 43 g

47. SPICY TOMATO BRUSCHETTA

Ingredients:
- One slice wheat bread
- One tablespoon Red Peppers Pesto Sauce
- One teaspoon olive oil
- One green tomato, sliced
- Dash dried pepper flakes
- Pinch of kosher salt
- Pinch of white pepper

Directions:
1. Spread pesto sauce on one side of the bread. Heat in the oven toaster.
2. Meanwhile, pour oil in a nonstick skillet set over medium heat. Saute tomatoes.
3. Transfer to a bowl. Season with dried pepper flakes, salt, and pepper. Spread mixture on bruschetta. Serve.

Nutritional Information
Calories: 110
Total Fat: 5 g
Total Carbohydrate: 17 g
Sugars: 7 g
Protein: 2 g
Sodium: 35 g

48. SPICY CUCUMBER AND TOMATO BRUSCHETTA

Ingredients:

- One slice wheat bread
- One tablespoon Red Peppers Pesto Sauce
- One teaspoon olive oil
- One green tomato, sliced
- One cucumber, sliced
- Dash dried pepper flakes
- Pinch of kosher salt
- Pinch of white pepper

Directions:

1. Spread pesto sauce on one side of the bread. Heat in the oven toaster.
2. Meanwhile, pour oil in a nonstick skillet set over medium heat. Saute tomatoes.
3. Transfer to a bowl and tip in cucumber. Season with dried pepper flakes, salt, and pepper. Spread mixture on bruschetta. Serve.

Nutritional Information

Calories: 97
Total Fat: 4 g
Total Carbohydrate: 13 g
Sugars: 5g
Protein: 4 g
Sodium: 28 g

49. Spicy Bruschetta with Red Peppers and Spinach

Ingredients:

- One slice wheat bread
- One tablespoon Red Peppers Pesto Sauce
- One teaspoon olive oil
- One green tomato, sliced
- One cucumber, sliced
- One spinach, torn
- Dash dried pepper flakes
- Pinch of kosher salt
- Pinch of white pepper

Directions:

1. Spread pesto sauce on one side of the bread. Heat in the oven toaster.
2. Meanwhile, pour oil in a nonstick skillet set over medium heat. Saute tomatoes.
3. Transfer to a bowl and tip in cucumber and spinach. Season with dried pepper flakes, salt, and pepper. Spread mixture on bruschetta. Serve.

Nutritional Information

Calories: 110
Total Fat: 5 g
Total Carbohydrate: 17 g
Sugars: 7 g
Protein: 2 g
Sodium: 35 g

50. TOMATO SALAD SANDWICH

Ingredients:

- One slice toasted wheat bread
- One tablespoon Red Pepper-Walnut Pesto Sauce
- extra virgin olive oil, for drizzling
- Two cherry tomato, unripe, quartered
- Two red cherry tomatoes, cut
- ¼ teaspoon apple cider vinegar
- ¼ teaspoon balsamic vinegar
- pinch palm sugar, crumbled
- pinch of kosher salt
- pinch of white pepper

Directions:

1. Spread pesto sauce on one side of the bread. Heat in the toaster oven.
2. **Meanwhile, in a bowl, mix olive oil, cherry tomatoes, apple cider vinegar, balsamic vinegar, sugar, salt, and pepper. Mix well. Spread mixture on bread. Serve.**

Nutritional Information

Calories: 78
Total Fat: 4 g
Total Carbohydrate: 12 g
Sugars: 8 g
Protein: 1 g
Sodium: 31g

CHAPTER 4:BREAD SPREADS AND TOPPINGS

51. CROSTINI WITH AVOCADO AND TOMATO

Ingredients:
- Two slices wheat bread, toasted
- Two garlic cloves, peeled
- Pinch of Spanish paprika

For the avocado salad
- Two tablespoons lemon juice, freshly squeezed
- ½ avocado, minced
- Two sprigs cilantro, minced
- One ripe tomato, minced
- One leek, minced
- Pinch of sea salt
- Pinch of white pepper

Directions:
1. Preheat the oven toaster. Rub garlic cloves on both sides of the bread.
2. Meanwhile, combine lemon juice, cilantro, tomato, leek, sea salt, and pepper. Mix and mash. Adjust seasoning.
3. **Spread equal portions on bread slices. Place in the oven toaster to warm through. Sprinkle with paprika. Serve.**

Nutritional Information
Calories: 134
Total Fat: 8 g
Total Carbohydrate: 19 g
Sugars: 9 g
Protein: 3 g
Sodium: 23 g

52. CROSTINI WITH OLIVES AND ONIONS

Ingredients:

- Two slices wheat bread, toasted
- Two garlic cloves, peeled
- 1/8 teaspoon extra virgin olive oil

For the Vegetable Spread

- One teaspoon apple cider vinegar
- One large black olive in oil, thinly sliced
- One roasted red pepper in oil, julienned
- One green olive in brine, thinly sliced
- 1/8 cup onion, minced
- 1/4 cup cucumber, julienned
- Pinch of sea salt
- Pinch of black pepper

Directions:

1. Preheat the oven toaster. Rub garlic cloves on the toasted bread. Set aside.
2. In a bowl, combine apple cider vinegar, olive in oil, red pepper in oil, olive in brine, onion, cucumber, salt, and pepper. Adjust seasoning.
3. Spread on bread slices. Place in the oven toaster to warm through. Drizzle in olive oil. Serve.

Nutritional Information

Calories: 110
Total Fat: 5 g
Total Carbohydrate: 17 g
Sugars: 7 g
Protein: 2 g
Sodium: 35 g

53. CROSTINIWITH MUSHROOMS AND PARSLEY

Ingredients:
- Two slices wheat bread, toasted
- Two garlic cloves, peeled

For the toppings:
- Two tablespoons ghee
- Two tablespoons olive oil
- Four porcini mushrooms, thinly sliced
- One tablespoon lemon juice, freshly squeezed
- ¼ cup fresh parsley, minced
- Pinch of sea salt
- Pinch of white pepper

Directions:
1. Rub garlic cloves on the toasted bread. Set aside.
2. Meanwhile, in a skillet, pour oil and ghee. Tip in mushrooms for 4 minutes or until golden brown.
3. Pour lemon juice and parsley. Season with salt and pepper. Adjust seasoning.
4. **Spread on bread slices. Place in the oven toaster to warm through. Serve.**

Nutritional Information
Calories: 67
Total Fat: 9 g
Total Carbohydrate: 16 g
Sugars: 9 g
Protein: 5 g
Sodium: 29 g

54. Crostini with Smoked Salmon

Ingredients:

- Two slices wheat bread, toasted
- Two garlic cloves, peeled
- Four smoked salmon slivers
- Two sprigs fresh chives, minced

For the cucumber-capers spread

- One tablespoon capers
- ¼ cup tomatoes, minced
- ½ cup cucumbers, minced
- Pinch of sea salt
- Pinch of white pepper
- Two tablespoon lemon juice, freshly squeezed

Directions:

1. Preheat the oven toaster. Rub garlic cloves on the toasted bread. Set aside.
2. In a small bowl, combine salmon, capers, tomatoes, cucumbers, salt, and pepper. Adjust seasoning.
3. Spread on bread slices. Place in the oven toaster to warm through. Garnish with chives and sprinkle lemon juice. Serve.

Nutritional Information

Calories: 110
Total Fat: 5 g
Total Carbohydrate: 17 g
Sugars: 7 g
Protein: 2 g
Sodium: 35 g

55. CROSTINIWITH TOMATOES

Ingredients:

- Two slices wheat bread, toasted
- Two garlic cloves, peeled
- ⅛ teaspoon extra virgin olive oil

For the Tomato Spread

- Two teaspoons lemon juice, freshly squeezed
- One fresh oregano leaf, julienned
- One green tomato, minced
- 1 red tomato, minced
- Pinch of sea salt
- Pinch of white pepper
- Cayenne powder, optional

Same cooking procedure as Crostini with Chicken and Cashew

Nutritional Information

Calories: 87
Total Fat: 6 g
Total Carbohydrate: 12g
Sugars: 8 g
Protein: 9 g
Sodium: 12 g

Chapter 5: Easy Pick Me Ups

56. Lemon-Strawberry Pudding

Ingredients:

- 3 eggs
- Nonstick cooking spray
- 1 cup strawberry
- Two tablespoons maple syrup
- Two teaspoons lemon peel, shredded
- ¼ cup all-purpose flour
- ¼ teaspoon salt
- Three tablespoons lemon juice
- 1 cup fat-free milk
- Three tablespoons vegetable spread

Directions:

1. Coat slow cooker with cooking spray. Place the berries and pour maple syrup.
2. Meanwhile, in a bowl, combine maple syrup, lemon peel, flour, and salt. Add lemon juice, milk, and vegetable oil spread. Mix using an electric mixer until well combined. Set aside.
3. In another bowl. Whisk egg whites until soft peaks form. Pour batter over the berries.

   4. Cover and cook on high for 2 hours. Cool, uncovered for 1 hour. Serve.

Nutritional Information

Calories: 110
Total Fat: 5 g
Total Carbohydrate: 17 g
Sugars: 7 g
Protein: 2 g
Sodium: 35 g

57. LEMON-BLUEBERRY PUDDING

Ingredients:

- 3 eggs
- Nonstick cooking spray
- Two tablespoons maple syrup
- 1 cup blueberry
- Two teaspoons lemon peel, shredded
- ¼ cup all-purpose flour
- ¼ teaspoon salt
- Three tablespoons lemon juice
- 1 cup fat-free milk
- Three tablespoons vegetable spread

Directions:

1. Coat slow cooker with cooking spray. Place the berries and pour maple syrup.
2. Meanwhile, in a bowl, combine maple syrup, lemon peel, flour, and salt. Add lemon juice, milk, and vegetable oil spread. Mix using an electric mixer until well combined. Set aside.
3. In another bowl. Whisk egg whites until soft peaks form. Pour batter over the berries.
4. Cover and cook on high for 2 hours. Cool, uncovered for 1 hour. Serve.

Nutritional Information

Calories: 95
Total Fat: 8 g
Total Carbohydrate: 9 g
Sugars: 7 g
Protein: 8 g
Sodium: 12 g

58. FROZEN YOGURT WITH BLUEBERRIES, BANANA, AND PEACHES

Ingredients:
- One tub Greek yoghurt, low fat
- 1 cup fresh blueberries
- One banana, diced
- One peach, diced

Directions:
1. In a bowl, fold blueberries, banana, and peach into yoghurt. Mix until well combined. Divide into equal portions.
2. Scoop portions in small containers.
3. Freeze for 5 hours before consuming. Serve.

Nutritional Information
Calories: 110
Total Fat: 5 g
Total Carbohydrate: 17 g
Sugars: 7 g
Protein: 2 g
Sodium: 35 g

59. FROZEN YOGURT WITH STRAWBERRIES, KIWI, AND APPLE

Ingredients:
- One tub Greek yoghurt, low fat
- 1 cup fresh strawberries
- One kiwi, diced
- One apple, diced

Directions:
1. In a bowl, fold strawberries, kiwi, and apple into yoghurt. Mix until well combined. Divide into equal portions.
2. Scoop portions in small containers.
3. Freeze for 5 hours before consuming. Serve.

Nutritional Information
Calories: 99
Total Fat: 6g
Total Carbohydrate: 9 g
Sugars: 6 g
Protein: 3 g
Sodium: 14g

60. FROZEN YOGURT WITH GRAPES, CRANBERRIES, AND MELON

Ingredients:

- One tub Greek yoghurt, low fat
- 1 cup fresh grapes
- 1 cup cranberries
- One melon, diced

Directions:

1. In a bowl, fold raisins, cranberries, and watermelon into yoghurt. Mix until well combined. Divide into equal portions.
2. Scoop portions in small containers.
3. Freeze for 5 hours before consuming. Serve.

Nutritional Information

Calories: 110
Total Fat: 5 g
Total Carbohydrate: 17 g
Sugars: 7 g
Protein: 2 g
Sodium: 35 g

CONCLUSION

Thank you for purchasing this cookbook it is my sincere hope that you will apply the acquired knowledge productively.It's time to take control and start making our own sweet and delicious diabetic delights.

With recipes for all occasions or seasons, ranging from the perfect-for-winter. For those who are suffering from diabetes here are the best dessert recipes that can be found. Join me on a sweet, creamy, crunchy, and often sticky journey to discover your inner cook and to create some downright delicious diabetic recipes.